I'm Not Seventy

Female Edition

Jean Dawn Leigh

jadie
BOOKS

Published by
Jadie Books Limited 2007

Copyright © Jean Dawn Leigh 2007

ISBN 978 0 9549354-8-1

Cover illustration by Ian West

Typesetting by Jake Adie

Printed & bound by
York Publishing Services Ltd
64 Hallfield Road
Layerthorpe
York
YO31 7ZQ

This book is sold subject to the condition that it shall not, in any circumstances, be lent, resold, hired out or otherwise circulated without the publisher's prior consent in any form of binding or cover other than that in which it is published and without a similar condition including this condition being imposed on the subsequent purchaser.

For the not so young,
not so middle-aged,
not so sure

Other Not Really Titles

I'm Not Really 18 (female edition)

I'm Not Really 18 (male edition)

I'm Not Really 30 (female edition)

I'm Not Really 30 (male edition)

I'm Not Really 40 (female edition)

I'm Not Really 40 (male edition)

I'm Not Really 50 (female edition)

I'm Not Really 50 (male edition)

I'm Not Really 60 (female edition)

I'm Not Really 60 (male edition)

I'm Not Really 70 (male edition)

I'm Not Really Pregnant

I'm Not Really Getting Married

I'm Not Really Moving House

I'm Not Really Retiring

It's Not Really Christmas

Me, Seventy?

What is this world coming to? Whatever will they think of next? Really, this is the kind of thing that makes my blood boil. Oh, I apologise, you must be wondering what on Earth I'm ranting on about. Do forgive me, please. But, you see, by some strange combination of events, I seem to be travelling headlong towards a seventieth birthday. Seventieth! As in septuagenarian. Me! Have you ever heard of anything so ridiculous? There has clearly been a mistake somewhere. But I'm having a devil of a time trying to work out what I am going to do about it. Really I am. I

Me, Seventy?

mean, how can I be expected to explain to all my well-meaning family members and friends that it has absolutely nothing to do with me and that it would be quite wrong, fraudulent even, for me to even think about accepting greetings cards? Or presents? At my age! All right, all right, I know I've had a considerable

I'm Not Really Seventy

number of birthdays already. Very well, sixty-nine to be precise, but that really doesn't have very much to do with it. Nothing at all if the truth be known. You see, the simple fact of the matter is that I'm just not old enough to be seventy. Not remotely. Listen, I've been around long enough to know what an SYO

Me, Seventy?

looks like. Goodness me, I've seen hundreds of them in my time. They've been around for as long as I have. In fact, I wouldn't be surprised if some of them were well into their eighties, or even nineties, by now. Or huddled up in a corner of a communal residents' lounge in one of those preposterous (nobody) care(s) homes. Oh no, no, no, you can take my word for it, I promise you, I do not resemble them in any way whatsoever. And even if it were to be true, I'm just not prepared for such an event. You can't expect a youthful, sixty-something, trendy-looking, forward-thinking girl like me, all of a sudden, to metamorphose into a decrepit, fumbling, old Zimmer-frame-dependent individual overnight, can you? It just doesn't bear thinking about. So, whoever's bright idea this was to include me in their ranks had better think again. And make it quick because I am simply not prepared to entertain the matter. Not in any shape or form. Certainly not like Brenda next door who seemed perfectly at ease when it was her turn a few months ago. Took it on the chin. Appeared to enjoy it, even. But then, and you will promise not to repeat a word of this, please, she does, sort of, well, you know, look the part. I could see for a good few months that it was about to happen to her at any time. Kind of vocational, if you like. Aspirational even. Oh God, the poor dear. What must she think of me? Probably hopelessly jealous. Has seemed terribly off-hand lately, come to think of it. Who knows? Mind you, could simply be the onset of . . . oh dear, what is it with my memory these days? It's on the tip of my tongue. Begins with an 'e' or is it an 'a'? Anyway, you know, that condition they have when they just can't recall things. Poor Brenda. However, mustn't criticize, what is it they say, 'there but for the grace of God and all that'? Mind you, I shouldn't overly worry

Me, Seventy?

about the whole ghastly business because anyone will know my true age simply by taking a look at the way I choose my . . .

Clothes

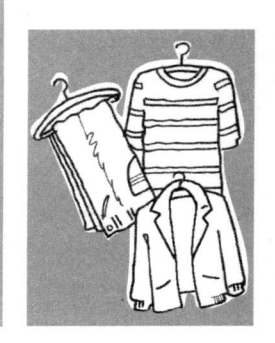

Well, it will be perfectly plain that my considerable wardrobe of high fashion items would be totally out of place in an SYO's home. Really, those poor old dears would think they'd been dressed up for the catwalk if they found themselves dolled up like me. But then, even though I say it myself,

Clothes

I've always had a particularly keen eye for what looks right on a woman. You know, the art of choosing the right costume for the right occasion. That indefinable something special. And without wishing to blow my own trumpet, most of those around me have always recognised the fact. For as long as I can remember eyes have invariably been cast in my direction whenever I've left the house sporting something new. Most people find it difficult not to just stare in total amazement. Can be quite off-putting, I can tell you – being regarded as a trendsetter as soon as I so much as step outside the front

Clothes

door. And that's not all. A quick glance at my present collection will reveal a positive leaning towards quality as well as style. And this is not some silly, passing fad of mine. No, no, no, my latest collection has taken years and years to acquire. Gosh, now let me think, yes, some of the items probably go back to before the war. And top quality they are too. Not like the flimsy, foreign-made rubbish the youngsters spend their money on these days. Well, really, you have to feel sorry for them, don't you. Last no time at all. You might find this difficult to believe but I've actually seen quite expensive garments so poorly put

Clothes

together that they're beginning to fall apart before they've even left the shops. Honestly. You mark my word, a new ladies outfitter's not far from here has rack upon rack of those blue, heavy-duty, cotton slacks with the knees already through. They're even displaying them on their mannequins in the shop window. And if they're not worn through and fraying, the dyes are so faded that they're fit only for a pauper. It just isn't good enough, I mean, what choice do the poor youngsters these days have of presenting themselves in a respectable manner? Before they've had a chance to leave the shop they

Clothes

find themselves looking like ragamuffins. It simply shouldn't be allowed. It's utterly preposterous – there should be a law against it. But then, I shouldn't concern myself unduly, it's for them to make a fuss in the same way that I would have done when I was their age. And talking of age, have you ever stopped to

consider what it
is with SYOs
and . . .

Memory?

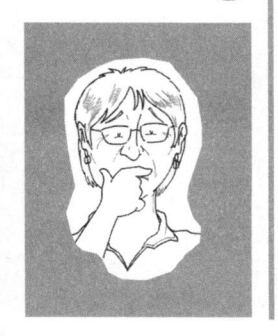

You won't need me to explain the difference between a typical SYO and a mere youngster like me where the subject of memory is concerned, I promise you. Yes, I'm fully aware that it's a terribly sad state of affairs for those who may have spent long and fulfilling lives, often holding down quite responsible posts in large organisations to suddenly find themselves at a loss to recall the simplest of events. But that is the way things are. The way the Good Lord planned them and who are we to object to His methods? If that is what He deems appropriate once mankind progresses to its

Memory?

twilight years then it's good enough for me. And, though I say it myself, once my mind is ready to accept that I am a fully-fledged septuagenarian then I will welcome the whole gamut of characteristics judged fit for a person of such senior years by the Great Maker in the sky. You see, the matter of memory loss is not just some random breakdown of faculties that develops the moment one's eighth decade appears on the horizon. No, of course it's not. He simply doesn't work that way. Each and every detail of the way we function is designed to the nth degree with a definite purpose to every last little twist

Memory?

and turn along the way. Well look at it like this. Why would an SYO need to remember anything like the number of events as efficiently as, say, a twelve-year-old? Mmm? Think about it. What items does a twelve-year-old have to remember to function as an effective twelve-year-old? Do you follow me? It's perfectly plain, isn't it? There are, of course, a million-and-one things she needs to recall to merely get through an ordinary day. Let me give you some 'for instances': Where did I leave my homework? What time do I need to get up to help mother polish the brass? Do my socks need darning?

Memory?

What lessons do I need to attend today? Have I pleated my skirt? Just to mention a few. There is no getting away from the fact that a twelve-year-old's mind has to deal with no end of items every minute of the day. Items that are of no concern whatsoever to her great, great, SYO aunt. Her life just doesn't bear any resemblance to that of an SYO. I mean, even a relative youngster like me has more on her plate to contend with what with the busy social life I lead: helping out in the local charity shop, village hall jumble sales and . . . er, well, there must be other things even if they don't come readily to mind. But my point is .

Memory?

. . you know . . . what I'm trying to say is that, well . . . now where exactly was I? Oh yes, twelve-year-olds, the fact of the matter is, they have lots more to think about than the old'uns. Far more things. Like, where they left their homework and whether their socks might need darning, for example. Things like that. And, well, there must be lots of other things like, well, it's difficult for me to just come up with them on the spur of the moment but you understand the point I'm trying to make surely. I mean, it's obvious, don't you think? People such as twelve-year-olds and me have a far greater need for instant recall. It's what distinguishes us

Memory?

from SYOs. In a way, it's not at all unlike . . .

Music

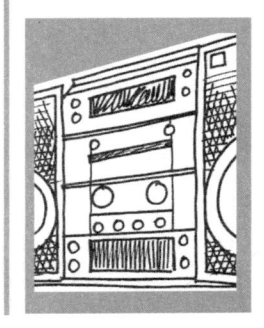

I mean the sort of music ordinary people listen to compared to SYOs. Now please don't think I'm being unduly critical or judgemental about the poor old souls artistic leanings. No, far be it for me to cast myself as the arbiter of good taste although I'm as qualified as any even if I do say it myself. Anyway,

Music

be that as it may, it has nothing to do with the point I am making. Which is, simply, that for those brought up during a time when the choice was either high-brow orchestral or low-brow music hall the opportunity to develop, how can I say it?, a sophisticated ear, was just not an available option. Nothing to do with them, you understand. The poor things were merely victims of the age they found themselves born into. And you can hardly blame a society whose young, otherwise highly-creative and artistic folk were ravaged by four solid years of a mindless and relentless war defending the sovereignty of their

Music

homeland. If the best their popular offerings could do was recount the deliberations of a certain young lady whose husband recommended that she should do her best to maintain a reasonable distance behind his vehicle without becoming distracted in the process then so be it. You have to take into account the fact that we more privileged folk are able to freely enjoy a wide range of musical styles whose composers and performers are inordinately uninhibited by such cultural restrictions. Not to mention the modern, highly technological means through which we are able to listen to our favourite

Music

tunes. Gone are the days of the wind up gramophone. My God, can you imagine having to endure winding the damn thing up every time the music began to slow down and fade? The truth is we are now existing in the future and are surrounded by every possible gadget to aid our every whim. My, you wouldn't believe how wonderful it is for me to sit back in my favourite easy chair listening to the dulcet tones of Vera Lynn or Paul Robson on my collection of 78s. Mind you, I don't seem to have so many left these days. Seem to have broken or scratched so many and I can't find out where to buy any replacements.

Music

All the shops I've tried seem to be out of stock. The shopkeepers just raise their eyes to the heavens whenever I ask. It must be so frustrating for them, poor things. But then, I suppose that's the price you pay for keeping up to date. Everyone is buying the stocks up as soon as they're put on the shelves. Still, I mustn't complain — although I've not used it for ages, I can always resort to the good, old faithful wireless. I'll just have to make do tuning into the BBC Light Programme. That way I'll have all the very latest popular songs at my fingertips. Although I must say I've been having dreadful trouble tuning

Music

into my favourite stations lately. And I can't seem to find the BBC Home Service anywhere on the dial these days. Let's just hope the Light Programme is where it's always been. I don't know, anyone listening to me would think I'm an SYO myself what with all the problems I seem to be having. No, I shouldn't mock, one day I shall be their age and I certainly won't take kindly to hearing the young speaking ill of *my* generation then. It is our duty to show respect for those of more mature years even if we don't find it easy to understand their perspective on life. They come from a different time. A time when things were done

Music

differently. I mean, consider for a moment their view towards the subject of . . .

Sex

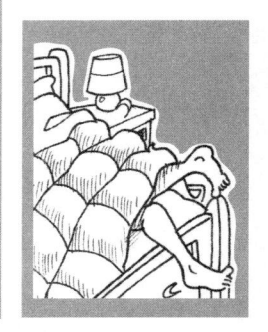

A subject our SYO friends would find extremely difficult to address, wouldn't you think? Seventy-year-olds and sex — the two just don't go together somehow, do they? Never did. Can't, for the life of me, imagine how they possibly produced another generation of

Sex

healthy human beings but that will just have to remain one of life's imponderables. A mystery that only the Good Lord has the answer to. Why he chose to design a generation looking like them is totally beyond me. A generation anyone in their right mind could not contemplate actually doing it, if you get my drift. Apart from the fact that neither gender could possibly want to, how would it be physically possible with all that arthritis? Not to mention replacement hips. And bi-focals for God's sake. A design fault if you ask me. I mean, most of them can hardly put one foot in front of the other let alone . . . well, I will have to leave the rest to your imagination. But you will see my point, surely? We're all girls of the world, are we not? And, as such, we know precisely how the Good Lord requires us to perform in order to secure the future of the species. Well, it's not so easy at the best of times, is it? All those arms and legs and dangly bits having to be arranged in the right order beneath a big heavy eiderdown and at least two layers of sheets and blankets. All tucked in, I'll have you! And, as if that's not enough, at night-time. With the electric light off! I mean, really, you can understand why even the best of us will get in a bit of a two-and-eight with all that to contend with, can't you? And then, when everything is finally in its designated place, the proceedings are expected to continue in a perfectly synchronised fashion. Not only without a word being uttered by either party but in the complete absence of anything remotely resembling a . . . well, a cue I suppose is what I've got in mind. All right, all right, I agree, a count of four would be ridiculous not to mention a metronome but you know what I'm getting at, it's all a bit much to expect even us youngsters to just fall into line and get it right every time, don't

Sex

you think? I mean, even a small musical ensemble would insist on establishing some form of tempo to ensure that all parties strike up at the same time to maintain a reasonably synchronized performance. And with the state of our poor, poor, SYOs' memory incapacities, unless they're at it every night, they won't stand a chance-in-a-million of remembering where everything goes anyway. Look, without wishing to appear irreverent or blasphemous even, He really must have been having a bad day when He designed them, eh? Can you imagine the trouble their teachers must

Sex

have had when they were at school? Goodness, gracious, me, the idea of addressing a whole classroom full of young SYOs must have been mind-numbing. I mean, their whole development must have placed such a strain on the country. And relationships, can you imagine? And marriage! The wedding night, for goodness' sake. Now, I'm not normally superstitious. Don't have any truck with all that silly supernatural, paranormal stuff – a lot of ballyhoo if you ask me. But when it comes to SYOs and reproduction, well, there is simply no other answer to it: that

Sex

story about the storks MUST be true. There can be no other explanation and that's all I'm prepared to say on the matter. I really must move on. There are so many other areas that will illustrate, most graphically, how I cannot possibly be ready to join the SYO ranks. For example, take the way they conduct a . . .

Conversation

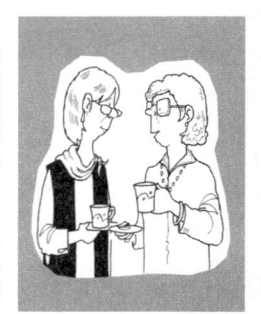

You must have witnessed that, surely. Two SYOs locked in dialogue with one another. One of the most baffling of life's experiences, I promise you. What could possibly drive them to participate in such an extraordinary, time-wasting exercise? There must, surely, be a hundred-and-one other things they could chose to engage in. If you've yet to have the privilege I'll let you in on some of the details. Right, where to start? Yes, imagine you're approaching a pair of them from some distance away. Nothing untoward; two seemingly normal individuals save for the obvious SYO deficiencies.

But when you begin to get within hearing range, things take on a whole new, somewhat curious perspective. What at first appeared to be perfectly plausible discourse between two mutually engaged members of the community now beggars belief. Let me give you an example of what might follow:

SYO1: "Have you seen Dotty lately?"

SYO2: "Oh yes, I've got them all over my left arm."

SYO1: "What's Dotty doing at the farm?"

SYO2: "I know, but if I don't keep calm they'll just keep spreading."

Do you see what I'm getting at? You've probably heard this kind of thing yourself, it's quite common these days. And, of course, very sad. But that's the sort of mess you get into when you've all but lost your hearing. Not as bad as losing it altogether, I'll grant you. When that happens there's no hope for any sort of

Conversation

social interaction. None at all. But when there's just a trace of a facility left you can literally chat away for hours without ever knowing anything is up. Honestly. And you'd think if our poor old SYO folk new anything about what was actually happening they'd save themselves an awful lot of time and effort by staying at home and talking to themselves. It'd be just as productive, don't you agree? But then, who are we to spoil their enjoyment? Not for us to dictate what our fellow folk should be doing with their lives. Live and let live, that's what I always say. Keeps you out of a lot of mischief that

Conversation

way. Treat others the way you'd wish them to treat you. Don't upset those around you even if you're sure they're in the wrong. Like the other day; there I was at home minding my own business when the telephone began to ring. Nothing unusual about that, I thought. No, but would you believe it?, there was a fellow on the other end of the telephone line who said he was from the local post office and that he wanted me to know that he had an under livid male for me. Fellow must have been positively out of his mind. I asked him what he thought he was doing, and that if the male he was ranting on about was, indeed, *under* livid then he should jolly well thank his lucky stars that the individual wasn't *over* livid at having to contend with a nincompoop like him in the workplace. I ask you, what is this world coming to? I mean, you'd think the Post Office would vet their staff more thoroughly to avoid upsetting good customers like me. Should have been sent to an asylum. Anyway, mustn't get too uptight, not good for the blood pressure. Now where was I? Oh yes, irrefutable reasons why you'll agree that I am simply worlds apart from our fellow SYO folk. Well, need we look further than the way an SYO views the subject of . . .

Politics

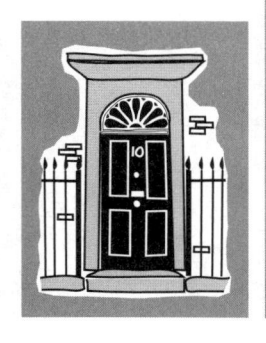

Now this one will make you laugh. Or, more likely, cry. Okay, I'll be honest here, politics is not something I profess to know an awful lot about. I'm not ignorant of the subject, I'll have you know, but it isn't, how can I put it?, the first on my list of priorities when, for instance, I open a newspaper. I certainly make it my business to keep abreast of most current topics as we all should otherwise how can any of us expect the country to be run the way we feel it should. Ostracise yourself from important social matters and you've only got yourself to blame when everything goes belly up. Well, that's my philosophy,

Politics

anyway. All right, I accept there are some complicated constitutional issues that are best left to the experts. Those who've spent years studying the subject and are in a position to grasp the intricacies involved. And it's right that we should rely upon them to represent us. And fight for our rights to ensure that other powers, be they neighbouring countries or parties within our own nation with dangerous, extreme agendas, are deterred from wantonly compromising the security for which our forefathers fought tooth and nail. Yes, the difficult issues have to be handled by those who know best.

Politics

But, of course, as we all know, there are all manner of topics that affect us on a daily basis that do not require the brains of Einstein to come to terms with. Like education and healthcare policies that are clearly at the root of a efficient and prosperous nation. Agree? Of course you do. I mean, what would be the point of our responsible, learned leaders placing all of their energies on foreign policy when our kids aren't being educated efficiently and our communities at large aren't receiving effective medication? Would be utterly nonsensical. So that's why it is incumbent upon the likes of you and me to take

Politics

an interest in basic issues to see that some toffee-nosed, old Etonian isn't just gallivanting around Westminster and putting himself first at the expense of the rest of us. There. I've said it. Got it off my chest. Mmm, and I feel a lot better for it, I can tell you. But, alas, we must return to our SYOs because, I'm afraid to say, their requirement for a government to hold office in the halls of Westminster with a workable majority of elected representatives from each of the six-hundred-and-however-many Great British regional constituencies would, if left to their devices, be solely dependant upon the

Politics

inclusion of a manifesto item promising to reduce the price of doctors' prescriptions by 2p. I know, I know, before you all get on your high horses, such a reduction is not, repeat, not to be sneezed at. This goes without saying. And we're all aware that living on a pension can be crippling at the best of times.

But come on, please. Any politically-aggressive, militant, authoritarian, fascist bunch of idiots prepared to put up a few thousand quid in an effort to recruit this society's ever-growing hooligan element with the promise of launching an immediate military assault on the European

Politics

mainland could, with no more than two minutes on the HQ word-processor, increase their popularity stakes fourfold by offering the old cronies tuppence. If it wasn't so funny we'd be scared out of our wits. It is, therefore, essential for each and every one of us to take a responsible attitude towards such matters and, although I might be stretching the remit of this communication somewhat, I would like to appeal to all of you of a similar youthful inclination to confront your local parties on the very issues that matter most: the sensible siting of speed cameras, regular wheelie bin collections

Politics

and more government subsidies for the arts, to name but a few. That way we'll effectively counter the inevitable wasted SYO votes. Now, if I have not convinced you of my total lack of an impending SYO status, then join me in taking a quick look at what a typical SYO will include in her list of . . .

Hobbies

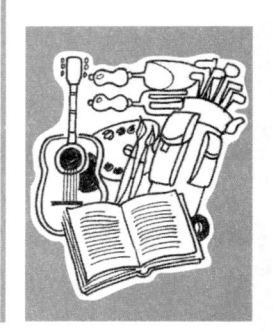

You know, things that make life that little bit more interesting. Things that give us a warm, comfortable feeling whenever we think about them. Because, without the prospect of involving ourselves with some all-consuming activity or other our days would be all the more dreary for it. And if you're like

Hobbies

most of us, an avid interest first introduced early on in life may well form the basis of our most rewarding pastimes in these, how should I put it, more senior years? Before you get off on the wrong track, I'm not talking about highly energetic sport activities. Oh no, even an agile, relative youngster like me would be hard pressed to last more than fifteen minutes with a hockey stick in my hand. Or even more pedestrian pursuits such as table tennis or bicycling into town on a windy afternoon. No, there is nothing wrong with admitting to oneself that certain activities are simply the preserve of the very young.

Hobbies

Nothing to be embarrassed or upset about. If nothing else, we must recognise our own capabilities and concentrate on what is befitting for our stage of life. So when I mention a bonding we may have been fortunate to have made many years ago, I'm referring to the types of things that are not dependent on our physical strengths and agilities. Like painting, playing music, writing poetry, etc. Activities such as these can be so mentally rewarding that a whole pattern of existence can quite easily be built around them. And one doesn't have to stop at following one's interest in isolation or, indeed, within the confines of

Hobbies

the home. No, there are all manner of clubs and societies within easy reach of all of us where these various disciplines can be developed. Often with the help of visiting professionals eager to impart their knowledge to the less informed amongst us. And it doesn't need to stop there. A whole social environment can be easily established with local, like-minded folk to provide a rich and fulfilling network of friends and acquaintances able to provide each other with a constant stream of support and stimulation. This is what helps make our lives so satisfying and rarely costs more

Hobbies

than a few pounds here and there for materials, maybe, or subscriptions to meet the moderate costs of hiring clubrooms etc. Yes, as far as I'm concerned, life would be very dull without them. But here, we must turn to our friends, the SYOs and ask where exactly do they fit in to the picture? Well, sadly, I have to report, not very favourably. If at all, in fact. The question is, what precisely do SYOs chose to involve themselves in to enrich their lives? Mmm, difficult. Well, almost impossible, if I'm to be truthful. The fact of the matter is, most of them spend the majority of their time complaining.

Hobbies

Yes, spouting off to all and sundry about how the world would be a better place if everyone did things their way. How the young people of today would benefit from conducting themselves in a manner popularised during the reign of Queen Victoria. How the new fangled this and that shouldn't be allowed. And all for one universally, all-encompassing reason: that things were simply done more efficiently, more tastefully, more intelligently, more respectfully and more anything-that-comes-to-mind in their day. The one and only activity that can possibly constitute a hobby: complaining.

Hobbies

Well, for all I care, they can complain for all they're worth. Nobody, but nobody can convince me that their times could hold a candle to mine. If the youngsters of today would care to stop for a moment and take a leaf out of my book the world would be all the better for it and I am simply not prepared to hear another word on the subject. I rest my case.